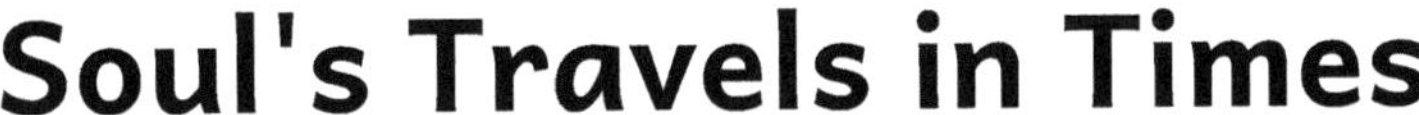

Soul's Travels in Times

Jack and Jill, both successful in their fields, had a romantic affair that led them to purchase a house in a leafy South London suburb. They dreamt of starting a family.

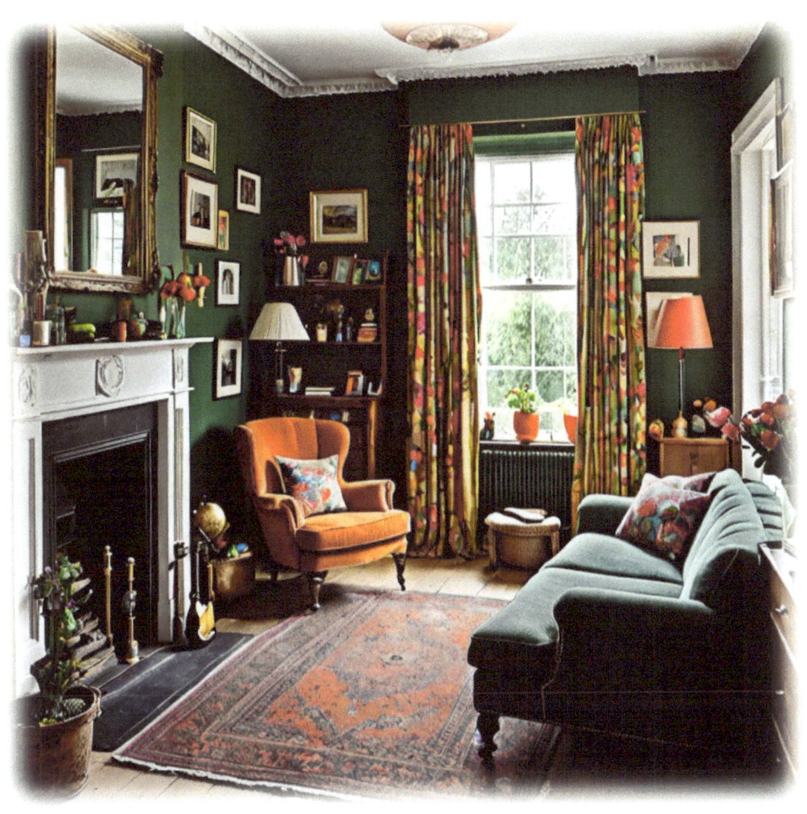

They tried for a year to conceive naturally, but their efforts bore no fruit. They decided to venture the path of IVF, choosing a highly re-garded clinic on Harley Street.

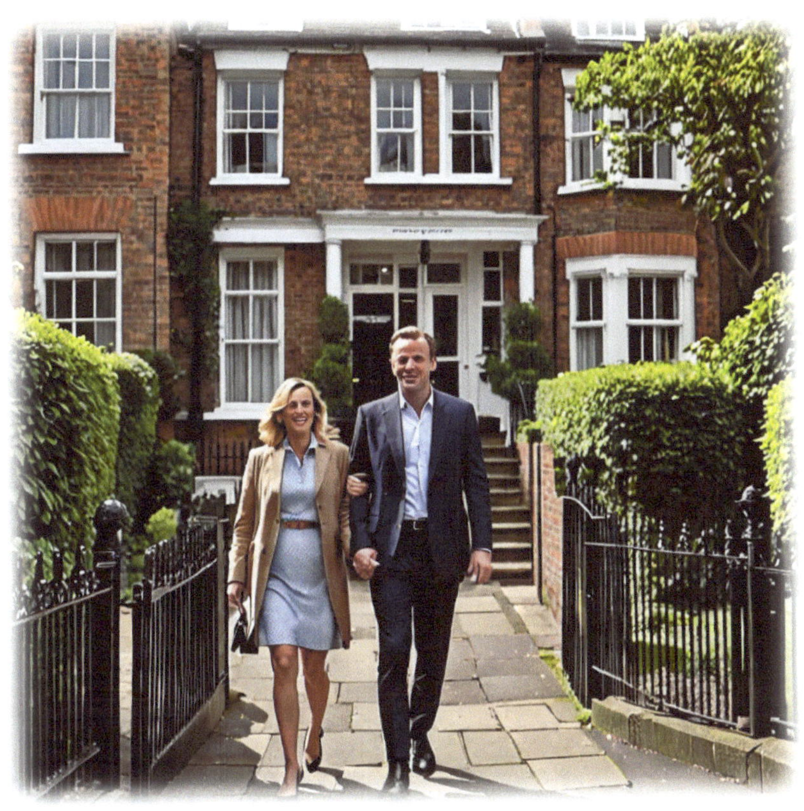

Three unsuccessful IVF rounds left them disheartened. They decided to turn towards a holistic approach, involving acupuncture, herbal teas, and spiritual retreats.

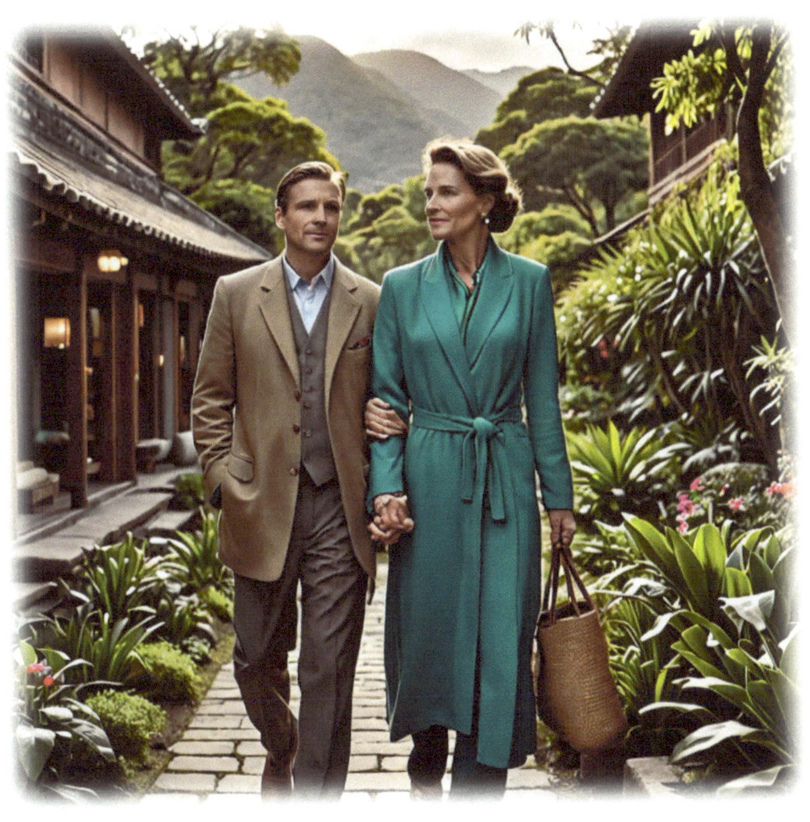

This path led them to discover their past lives through family constellations. They learned they were a couple in Germany during the Second World War, with a daughter who was torn from them.

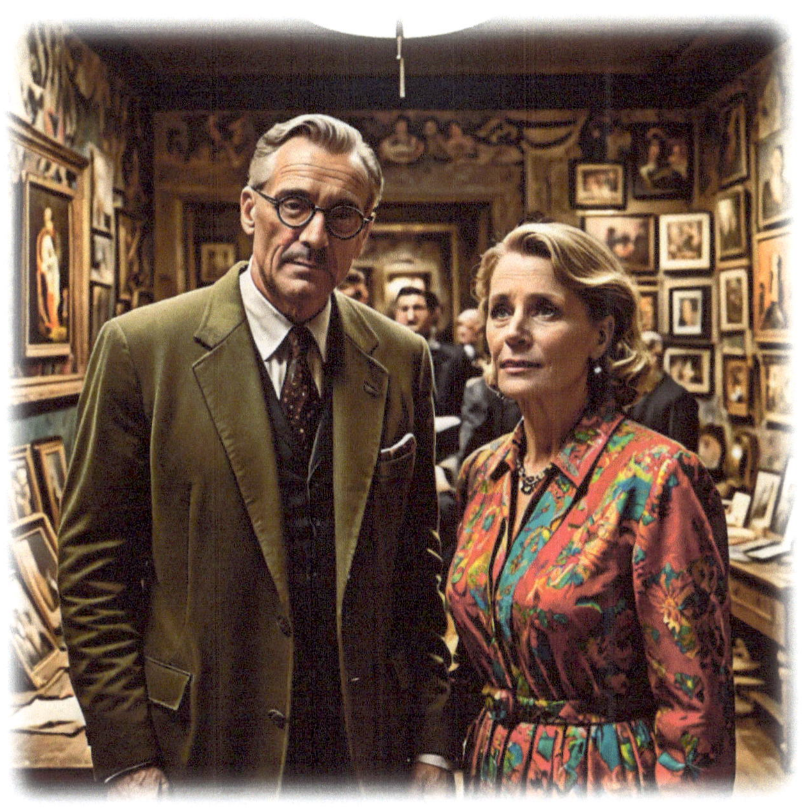

They spent a year exploring other IVF centres across the globe, hoping to find a solution. Meanwhile, their spiritual journey continued.

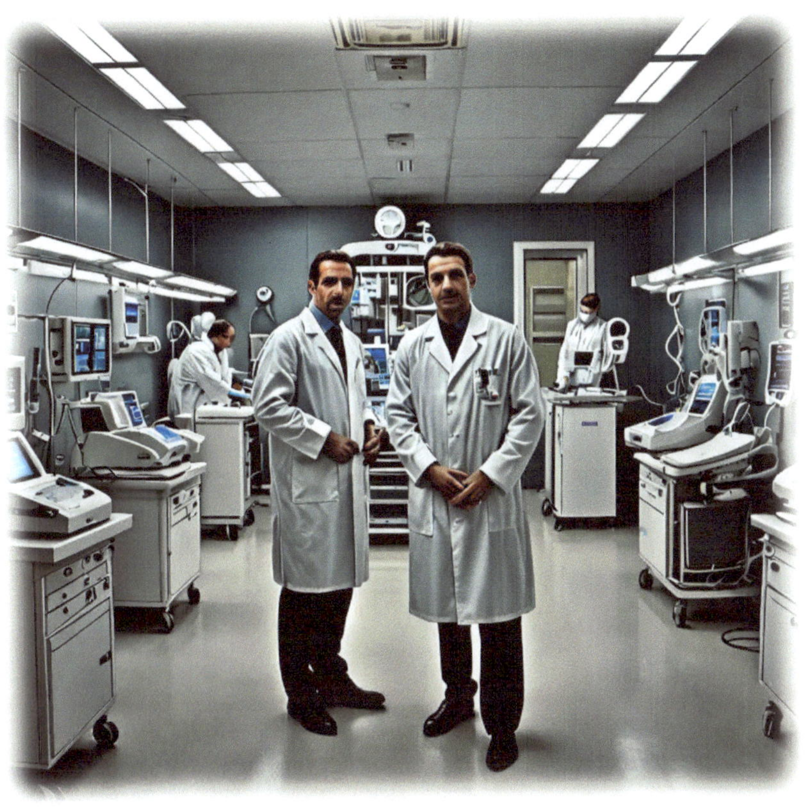

One evening in Istanbul, they met
a couple discussing soul journeys.
The conversation steered them towards visiting concentration cam-
ps, to connect with their past lives.

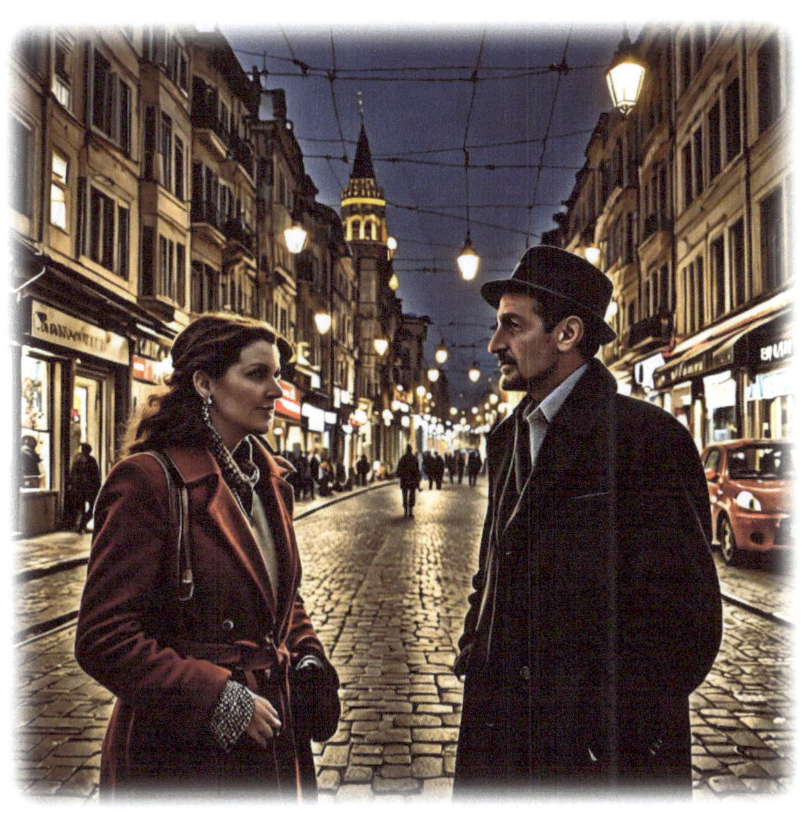

They visited Auschwitz,
Bergen-Belsen, Buchenwald, and
Flossenburg. Each visit brought
them closer to their past and helped
them reconcile with their fears.

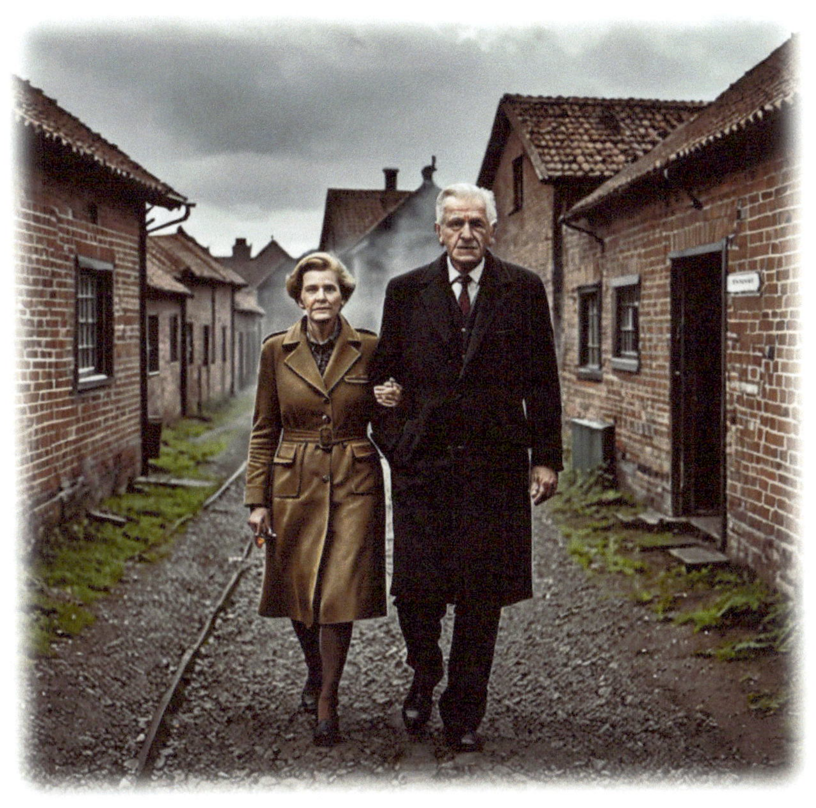

In Germany, they found a clinic that performed a myomectomy for Jill. This renewed their hopes of starting a family.

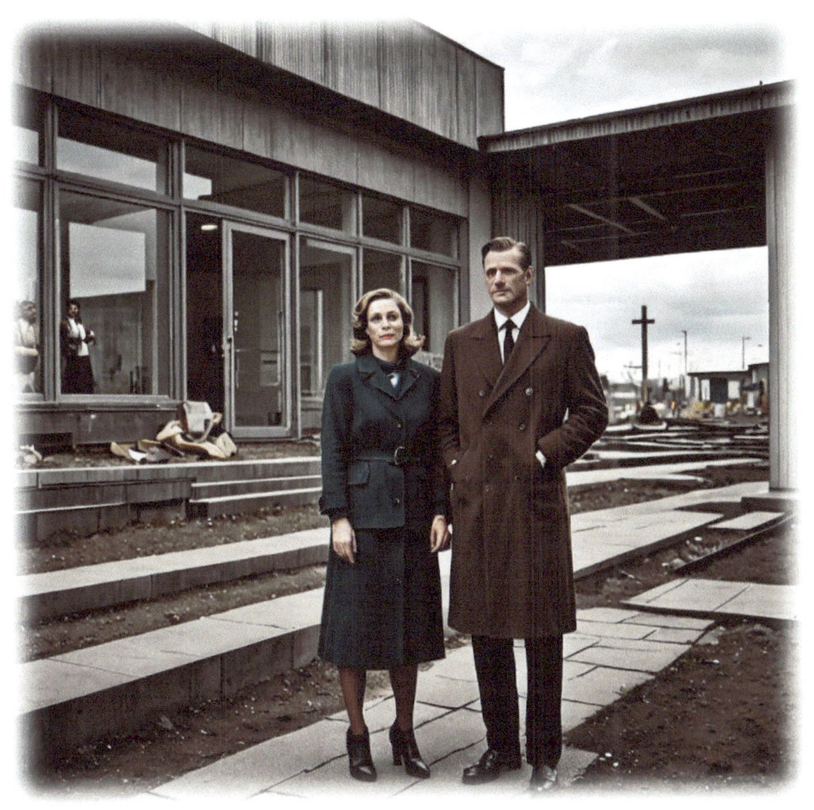

Jack surprised Jill with a romantic holiday to Malta. The trip was a breath of fresh air, an escape from the stress they had been under.

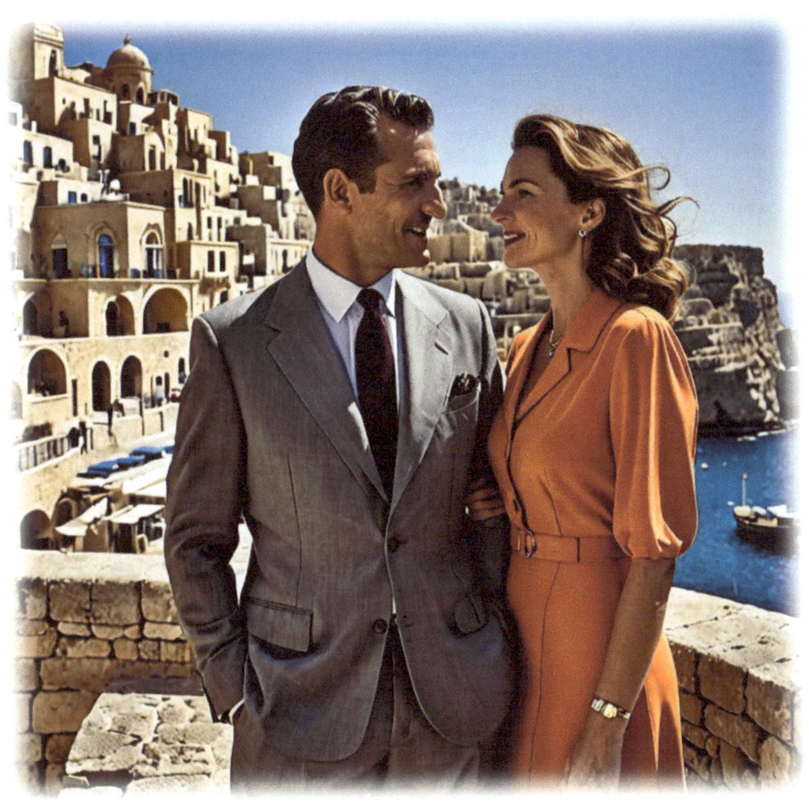

Shortly after their holiday, Jill dis-
covered she was pregnant. At the
age of 44, she was finally going to be
a mother. Their joy knew no bounds.

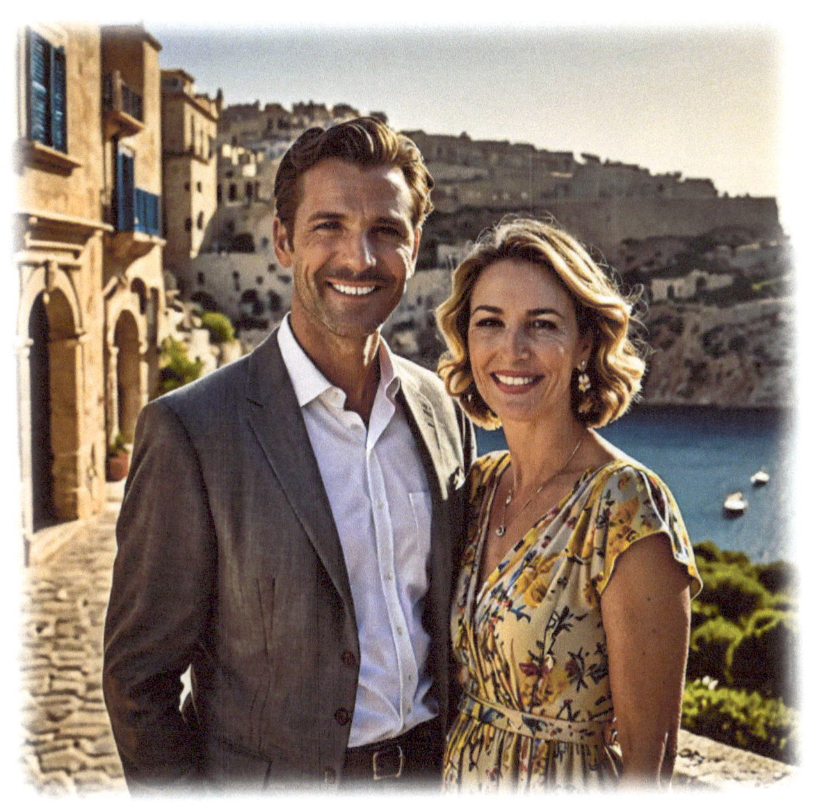

Jill gave birth to a healthy girl, whom they named Anna. Their journey, filled with trials and tribulations, had finally led them to their daughter.

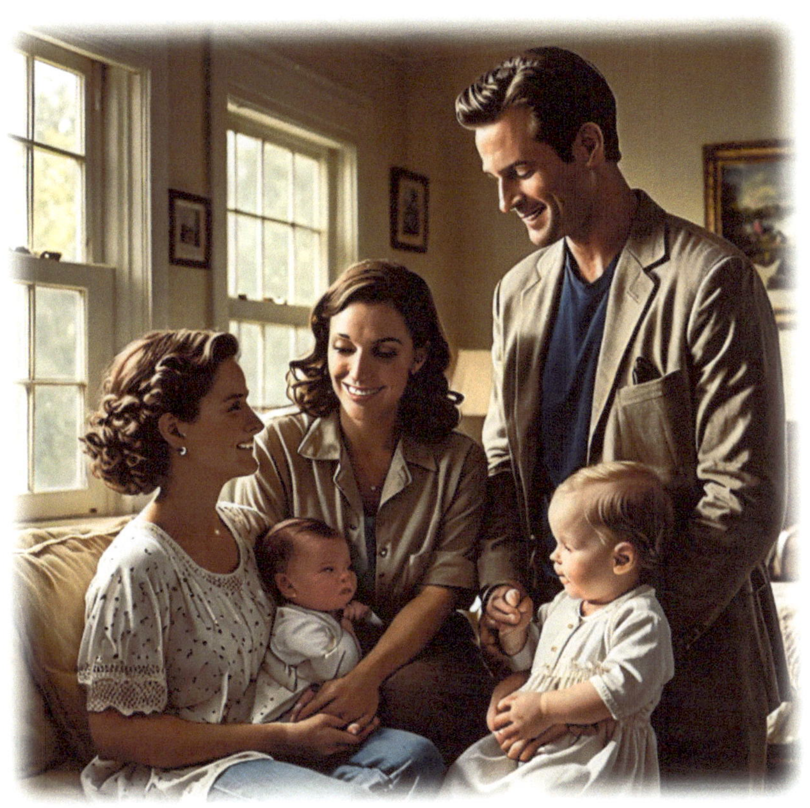

Jack and Jill learned that a child is born to continue a story between two people. Their story, and now Anna's, was a testament to love, perseverance, and the power of soul connections.

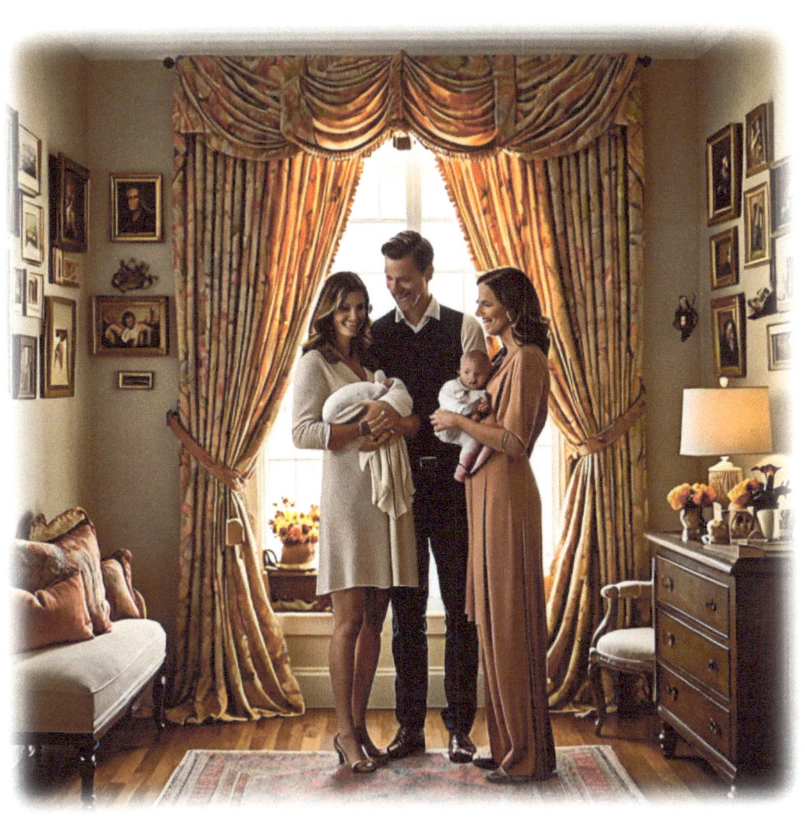

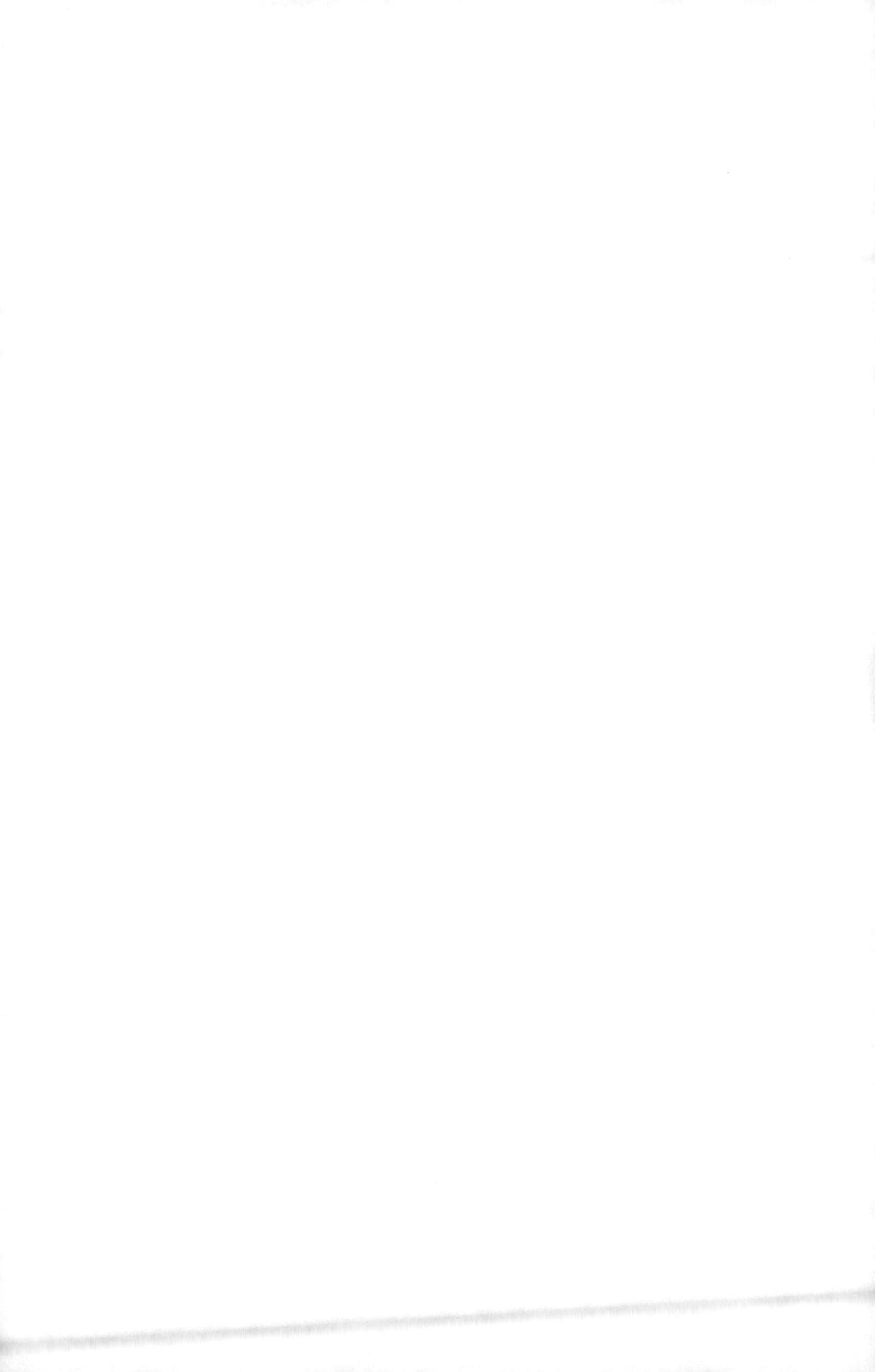

The End.